ISOMETRIC EXERCISE SECRETS FOR WOMEN

Your Workout Guide to Strengthening Your Core, becoming Fitter, Less Stressed, and Empowered

ISOMETRIC EXERCISE SECRETS FOR WOMEN

Your Workout Guide to Strengthening Your Core, becoming Fitter, Less Stressed, and Empowered

Amy Priolo

Table of Contents

Introduction

Tara believed in the benefits of movement and exercise, but her busy schedule made it tough to regularly visit the gym. Curious about isometric exercises, she decided to try them out to dispel myths surrounding this seemingly stationary fitness method.

Tara started adding isometric exercises to her daily routine. Initially, some doubted the effectiveness of these seemingly still movements. However, Tara persisted, focusing on muscle contractions without fancy equipment or intense cardio.

Over time, something magical occurred. Tara experienced a subtle but profound transformation in her body. Contrary to the misconception that isometric exercises were static and dull, Tara found a quiet beauty in their simplicity.

The myth that isometric exercises lacked intensity was shattered as Tara's muscles strengthened. Her arms, core, and legs improved without the need for vigorous movement. Isometric magic worked wonders beneath the surface, sculpting her body with grace that defied stereotypes.

Yet, the true beauty of Tara's isometric journey went beyond the physical. Amidst the stillness, she discovered mental clarity. Engaging in these exercises became a mindful practice, a serene moment in her day to connect with her body.

As weeks passed, Tara debunked more myths than she imagined. Isometric exercises weren't just for strength; they offered a holistic well-being approach. The idea that exercise had to involve complicated movements was replaced by the elegant simplicity of intentional positions.

Tara enjoyed benefits beyond the gym. Her joints felt stable, stress melted away during these mindful moments. The myth that isometrics were restrictive vanished as Tara seamlessly integrated them into different life phases, even during postpartum recovery.

One day, standing tall, feeling strength radiate through her, Tara realized isometric exercises had become her compass. They guided her toward a healthier, balanced life, proving that beauty and strength could emerge from intentional still movements. Tara's isometric journey testified to the transformative power of embracing a different fitness kind—going beyond myths and leaving her feeling beautifully empowered.

Introducing...Isometric Exercise Secrets for Women

Your Guide to a Stronger Core, Improved Fitness, Reduced Stress, and Empowerment

Embark on an exciting adventure with "Isometric Exercise Secrets for Women" – the key to unlocking your hidden strength and vitality. Immerse yourself in a world of fitness tips that promise not only physical changes but a complete renewal of your body, mind, and spirit.

Reasons to Explore this Guide:

1. Boost Your Core: Explore the hidden world of isometric exercises made to strengthen your core. See the magic happen as you shape a strong, resilient center that exudes confidence.

2. Revamped Fitness: Say goodbye to tiring workouts that take up your time and energy. Explore routines designed for today's busy woman – efficient, effective, and seamlessly fitting into your schedule.

3. Complete Transformation: Feel the harmony of isometrics and overall wellness. Enhance your fitness journey by gaining not just physical strength but mental peace. Embrace a life where strength, flexibility, and empowerment are intertwined.

4. Personalized Approach: Whether you're new to fitness or a seasoned enthusiast, learn to adjust isometric workouts to your liking. This guide is your guide, leading you through a personalized fitness adventure tailored to your goals.

5. Stress-free Empowerment: As isometric exercises reveal their secrets, find the path to a less stressed and more empowered self. This book is your guide to achieving not only physical strength but overall well-being.

6. Results Unfold: See your progress, celebrate achievements, and adjust goals on this transformative journey. "Isometric Exercise Secrets for Women" is not just a guide; it's your companion in the exciting quest to become the strongest, most empowered version of yourself.

Why Wait? Uncover the Secrets Today!

The time for change is now! Discover the tips, embrace the strength, and step into a future where you're not just fit – you're empowered. Dive into the pages of empowerment and let the path to your newfound strength commence! Your empowered future is just a read away!

Chapter 1: Introduction to Isometric Exercises

Let's begin by exploring isometric exercises designed for women in a scientific way. We will break down the details of isometric training, explaining its factual foundations and how it affects the body. Get ready to learn about static strength training, focusing on the simple but powerful principles that make it effective. Let's understand the basics of muscle contractions, unraveling the benefits that boost women's strength, resilience, and overall well-being. Welcome to a chapter grounded in facts, emphasizing the physiological aspects of isometric exercises.

Understanding Isometric Exercises

Isometric exercises, also called static strength training, involve muscle contraction without changing length. To put it simply, you're applying force without visible movement. While these exercises might not make you sweat like dynamic movements, they bring significant benefits, making them valuable in any fitness routine.

How Isometric Exercises Work

During an isometric exercise, muscles create tension, but there's no joint movement. Think about holding a plank – your muscles are working, your core is tight, but you're not actively moving. This sustained contraction builds strength by challenging muscles against resistance. The longer you hold, the more your muscles adapt and become stronger.

Targeting Specific Muscle Groups

Isometric exercises excel at effectively targeting specific muscle groups. Unlike traditional exercises engaging multiple muscles at once, isometrics allow isolation and focus on a particular area. This makes them great for sculpting and toning specific body parts, meeting individual fitness goals.

Adaptable to Any Fitness Level

Isometric exercises suit any fitness level, whether you're a beginner or experienced. You can adjust intensity by changing hold duration or resistance, making isometrics accessible for women of all ages and fitness backgrounds. It offers a low-impact yet highly effective workout option.

Benefits of Isometric Exercises

Now that we've touched on how isometric exercises work, let's explore their numerous benefits.

Strength Building without Equipment

Isometric exercises stand out for their simplicity. Many can be done without expensive gym equipment. Bodyweight exercises like wall sits, planks, and static lunges can be performed anywhere, making them a convenient option for busy women without access to a fully-equipped gym.

Improved Joint Stability

Isometric exercises enhance joint stability by strengthening surrounding muscles. This is particularly helpful for women, preventing injuries and easing joint pain, especially in areas like knees and hips. The static nature of these exercises enhances stability without high-impact movements.

Time-Efficient Workouts

In the busy daily routine, finding time for a workout can be tough. Isometric exercises offer a solution with their time-efficient nature. Engage multiple muscle groups in a single exercise, maximizing workout effectiveness in less time. A game-changer for women with busy schedules, prioritizing fitness without sacrificing time.

Benefits of Isometric Training for Women

Now that we've understood isometric exercises' basics, let's highlight why incorporating this method into your fitness routine can be a game-changer, especially for women.

Targeted Muscle Toning

Isometric exercises enable precise muscle targeting, excellent for women looking to tone specific body areas. Whether defining arms, tightening the core, or shaping legs, isometrics help achieve desired aesthetic goals.

Enhanced Core Strength

A strong core is vital for a healthy body. Isometric exercises, like planks and abdominal contractions, activate core muscles differently than traditional exercises. This focused engagement aids in a toned midsection, improved posture, reduced back pain, and enhanced stability – crucial for women's overall well-being.

Joint-Friendly Fitness

Isometric training benefits women with joint sensitivities. Unlike high-impact activities, isometric exercises are gentle on the joints, minimizing stress. Ideal for individuals dealing with conditions like arthritis or recovering from injuries.

Functional Strength for Daily Activities

Isometric exercises mimic static muscle contractions needed in daily activities. Whether lifting groceries, carrying a child, or sitting at a desk, these exercises contribute to functional strength, improving daily life movements.

Stress Reduction and Mental Well-being

Isometric exercises not only benefit physical health but also mental well-being. Their focused nature requires concentration and control, providing a mindful and meditative aspect to your workout routine. This mental engagement can be a powerful stress-reliever, promoting calmness and balance.

Empowerment through Independence

Isometric training empowers women by offering independent exercise. Whether at home, in a park, or during a lunch break, integrate isometric exercises into your day without relying on a gym or specialized equipment. This fosters self-sufficiency, allowing you to take charge of your fitness journey on your terms.

Adaptable to Life's Phases

Women experience various life phases, including pregnancy and postpartum recovery. Isometric exercises can be adapted to suit these phases, providing a safe and effective way to maintain strength and fitness. Always consult with a healthcare professional before starting or modifying any exercise routine, especially during significant life changes.

By incorporating these exercises into your routine, you're not just working on strength; you're investing in overall health, resilience, and mental well-being. Embrace the power of isometric training and discover how it can elevate your fitness journey to new heights.

Chapter 2: Isometric Fundamentals

Stripping away unnecessary embellishments, we delve into the core aspects of anatomy and physiology, dissecting the intricacies of muscle function. Through the lens of simplicity, we uncover the principles that govern isometric training, emphasizing tangible facts and straightforward insights. This lays the groundwork for a pragmatic exploration, offering a comprehensive understanding of the biological underpinnings and guiding principles that form the basis of an effective isometric training regimen tailored for women.

The Basics of Anatomy and Physiology in Isometric Training

Understanding the mechanics of muscles and how they respond to isometric training is essential for maximizing the benefits of your workout.

Let's start with the basics. Muscles are the powerhouse of movement, enabling us to perform daily activities and engage in various exercises. Within the muscular system, different types of muscles exist, including skeletal muscles, smooth muscles, and cardiac muscles. For isometric exercises, our primary focus is on skeletal muscles, the ones attached to our bones that control voluntary movements.

Now, let's delve a bit deeper into the structure of skeletal muscles. Envision each muscle as a bundle of muscle fibers. These fibers contain smaller units known as myofibrils, where the magic of muscle contraction occurs. The fundamental unit of contraction is the sarcomere, a repeating unit along the myofibril responsible for muscle shortening.

When you engage in isometric exercises, you activate your muscles without altering their length. In contrast to dynamic exercises that involve movement, isometrics entail static contractions, where muscles generate force but don't visibly change in length. Grasping this concept is pivotal to understanding the essence of isometric training.

Moving on to the physiology of muscle contraction, it's crucial to acquaint yourself with the neuromuscular junction. This is where nerves communicate with muscles. When you decide to flex a muscle during an isometric exercise, your brain sends signals through your nerves, triggering the release of neurotransmitters that stimulate muscle contraction.

Now, let's explore the role of blood flow and oxygen delivery during isometric exercises. As muscles contract, they temporarily compress blood vessels, reducing blood flow and causing a buildup of metabolic byproducts like lactic acid. This natural process contributes to the overall effectiveness of isometric exercises.

Understanding the energy systems at play is also vital. Isometric exercises primarily tap into the anaerobic energy system, which doesn't rely on oxygen. This system provides quick bursts of energy, making isometrics an efficient choice for short, intense workouts.

By acknowledging how muscles function at a fundamental level, individuals can better harness the benefits of isometric training. Get ready to engage your muscles intelligently and make the most of your workout routine by understanding the intricate dance between anatomy and physiology.

Exploring the Principles of Isometric Training

Having covered the foundational aspects of anatomy and physiology, it's now time to delve into the principles that make isometric training a dynamic and effective approach to enhancing strength and overall fitness.

Principle 1: Time under Tension

Isometric exercises revolve around holding a muscle contraction for an extended period, a concept known as time under tension (TUT). Unlike dynamic exercises where muscles contract and lengthen, isometrics focus on a sustained contraction, intensifying the engagement of muscle fibers. This prolonged tension triggers metabolic responses, promoting muscle growth and endurance.

Principle 2: Progressive Overload

To witness continuous improvement, it's crucial to progressively challenge your muscles. Progressive overload in isometric training involves gradually increasing the intensity or duration of your contractions. This could mean adding resistance if you're using props, or holding the contraction for a longer duration. By progressively overloading your muscles, you stimulate continuous adaptation, fostering strength gains over time.

Principle 3: Specificity of Training

Isometric exercises provide the opportunity to target specific muscles or muscle groups with precision. Whether you're aiming to tone your arms, strengthen your core, or enhance your leg muscles, specificity in training ensures you focus on the areas you want to improve. This targeted approach makes isometrics versatile, allowing you to tailor your routine to meet your unique fitness goals.

Principle 4: Mind-Muscle Connection

Connecting your mind with your muscles is a fundamental aspect of isometric training. By concentrating on the muscle you're engaging and maintaining mental awareness throughout the contraction, you enhance the effectiveness of the exercise. This mind-muscle connection not only improves the quality of your workout but also promotes better overall body awareness.

Principle 5: Rest and Recovery

Just like any other form of exercise, adequate rest and recovery are essential for optimal results. Isometric training induces micro-tears in muscle fibers, and they need time to repair and grow stronger. Be mindful of your body's signals, ensure proper sleep, and incorporate rest days into your routine to allow your muscles to recover fully.

Principle 6: Breathing Techniques

Proper breathing is often overlooked but plays a crucial role in isometric exercises. Maintain a controlled and steady breathing pattern during contractions to ensure a steady oxygen supply to your muscles. Deep breaths can also help you maintain focus and reduce unnecessary tension, allowing you to get the most out of each isometric hold.

Principle 7: Safety First

Lastly, always prioritize safety. Whether you're a beginner or an experienced fitness enthusiast, proper form is paramount. Ensure you're in a stable position, especially if performing standing or weight-bearing isometrics. Listen to your body, avoid overexertion, and consult with a fitness professional if you have any concerns about your form or suitability for specific exercises.

These principles form the bedrock of effective isometric training for women. By incorporating these into your routine, you'll not only strengthen your muscles but also empower yourself with a versatile and engaging approach to fitness. Embrace these principles, stay consistent, and enjoy the transformative benefits of isometric exercises on your journey to a stronger and healthier you!

Chapter 3: Getting Ready: Preparing for Isometric Workouts

Before we jump into the practical stuff, let's lay the groundwork. Checking how fit you are helps make your workout safe and effective. Also, setting up a good workout area makes sticking to this healthy practice easier. This chapter gives simple tips and steps to guide you through the start, providing a strong base for your isometric exercises. Now, let's talk about the practical things, understand your abilities, and set up a good space for your well-being.

Checking Fitness Levels

Starting isometric exercises is exciting, and the first step is to see how fit you are. This helps make a workout plan that suits your strengths and areas to improve.

Think about your overall health. Are there any health issues you need to be careful about? Isometric exercises are generally safe, but it's good to think about any health concerns you have. If you're not sure, talking to a healthcare professional is a good idea.

Now, let's break down the fitness check:

Cardio Health:

A strong heart is vital for overall fitness. Think about activities that make your heart beat faster. Can you climb stairs without feeling tired? Try a brisk walk or light jog for 10-15 minutes and see how your body reacts. This helps set a starting point for your heart fitness.

Strength and Muscle Endurance:

Strength is important for isometric exercises. Test your muscles with basic exercises like push-ups or squats. How long can you hold a plank? These simple tests show what your muscles can do and help you start at the right level.

Flexibility:

Flexibility is often forgotten but matters a lot. Try reaching for your toes or doing simple yoga poses.

Checking flexibility helps find areas that need attention and prevents injuries in different activities.

Balance and Coordination:

Isometric exercises need stability, so check your balance. Stand on one leg for 30 seconds and notice if you wobble. Try simple coordination exercises like marching in place. These checks give a good idea of your physical abilities.

Joint Health:

Think about your joints—they're crucial for movement. Notice any discomfort or stiffness in certain areas. It's important to choose exercises friendly to your joints and adjust your routine if needed.

This check isn't about comparing or judging but is a useful guide for your fitness journey. With this knowledge, you can plan isometric exercises that match your abilities and gradually improve as you get stronger. If any worries come up, talking to a healthcare professional ensures a safe and enjoyable fitness experience. Now that you've checked your fitness, let's move on to creating a safe workout space in section 3.2. Ready for the next step?

Building a Safe Workout Space

Now that you know your fitness levels and are ready for isometric exercises, the next important step is to create a safe workout space. Having an environment that helps you focus, stay safe, and be consistent is key to a successful isometric workout routine.

Here's a guide to help set up the perfect workout space:

1. Choose a Dedicated Area:

Pick a specific spot in your home for isometric workouts. It doesn't have to be big, but having a dedicated area makes it clear that it's time to exercise. Make sure it's well-ventilated and free from distractions.

2. Clear the Clutter:

Keep your workout space free of obstacles. Remove anything that could trip you up. A clean and organized area not only makes it safer but also lets you move easily during exercises.

3. Invest in Proper Flooring:

Think about the flooring in your workout area. If possible, choose a surface that gives a bit when you step on it. Exercise mats or foam flooring are great for protecting your joints during isometric exercises.

4. Good Lighting:

Having enough light is important for safety and focus. Natural light is best, but if that's not possible, get bright, energy-efficient lighting for your workout space. This not only helps you see better but also boosts your mood and motivation.

5. Ventilation:

Make sure there's good airflow in your workout space. Proper ventilation keeps you from getting too hot and helps you stay comfortable during exercises. If you're inside, open windows or use a fan to keep a pleasant temperature.

6. Mirror, Mirror on the Wall:

Having a mirror in your workout space can be helpful. It lets you check your form and posture, making sure you're doing each isometric exercise right. This visual feedback makes your workout more effective.

7. Gather Your Equipment:

Depending on the isometric exercises you're doing, get any needed equipment ahead of time. Whether it's resistance bands, dumbbells, or stability balls, having everything ready saves time and keeps your routine consistent.

8. Create a Positive Atmosphere:

Make your workout space personal. Add things that inspire and motivate you, like upbeat music, quotes, or your favorite workout gear. A positive atmosphere makes isometric exercises more enjoyable.

9. Establish a Routine:

Being consistent is important for any fitness journey. Set specific times for your isometric workouts and stick to your schedule. This not only helps make it a habit but also makes sure you set aside time for your health.

By creating a space that suits you, you make an environment where isometric exercises can work well. This careful approach makes sure you're safe, not distracted, and in a positive mindset during your workouts. Now that your workout space is ready, you're all set to start your isometric exercise routine with confidence. Excited to begin your workouts in this well-prepared space?

WHAT LESSONS HAVE YOU LEARNT SO FAR?

Chapter 4: Unveiling the Power of Isometric Exercises

Unlocking a stronger, more toned physique doesn't always demand constant motion; in fact, the secret may lie in the power of stillness. This chapter explores the fascinating world of isometric exercises specifically designed for women. Forget the misconception that fitness necessitates perpetual movement. Here, we present a detailed guide to sculpting robust shoulders, well-defined arms, powerful legs, and firm glutes—all through the art of holding steady. No need for intricate routines; just the simplicity of isometrics to spark transformative changes in your body. Get ready to embrace a fitness approach that demonstrates strength in the stillness of controlled contractions. Let's dive into the details!

Isometrics for the Upper Body

Let's delve into the essential aspects of upper body isometrics and understand how they can benefit you.

Building Strong Shoulders and Toned Arms

Shoulder Stability:

Begin work on your upper body by focusing on constructing robust and stable shoulders. Isometric exercises engage your shoulder muscles without the need for repetitive movements, making them ideal for joint-friendly workouts. An excellent exercise to achieve this is the isometric shoulder press.

Start by standing with your feet shoulder-width apart, holding a weight or resistance band at shoulder height. Push upwards against the resistance, engaging your shoulder muscles, and hold for a count of 10-15 seconds. This not only targets your deltoids but also enhances overall shoulder stability.

Toning Arms:

Moving on to the arms, isometric bicep and tricep exercises are exceptional for sculpting and toning without excessive bulk. Try the isometric bicep curl by holding a dumbbell in each hand, palms facing forward. Keep your elbows close to your body, curl the weights halfway up, and hold the position. This concentrates tension on your biceps, promoting muscle definition.

For triceps, the isometric tricep kickback is your go-to. Stand with a dumbbell in your right hand, hinge forward at the hips, and extend your arm back. Hold this position, feeling the burn in your triceps, and repeat on the other side. These exercises, with their static holds, effectively activate your muscles for a more toned and sleek appearance.

Sculpting Defined Back Muscles

A strong, defined back not only improves your posture but also contributes to an overall sculpted appearance. Isometric exercises provide an excellent means of achieving this, particularly with the isometric pull-up.

Using a sturdy horizontal bar, position your hands shoulder-width apart with palms facing away from you. Jump up, then slowly lower yourself halfway down and hold for as long as you can. This targets your latissimus dorsi and rhomboid muscles, fostering a well-defined and toned back.

Additionally, the isometric row is fantastic for targeting your middle and upper back muscles. Using resistance bands or weights, hinge at your hips and pull the resistance towards your chest, holding for several seconds. This not only improves your back muscles but also engages your core for added benefits.

Incorporating these upper body isometric exercises into your routine will not only strengthen and tone your shoulders and arms but also contribute to an overall balanced physique. Consistency is key, so make these exercises a regular part of your fitness routine for lasting and noticeable results.

Isometrics for the Lower Body

Let's now check out a variety of isometric exercises focusing on building powerful legs and sculpting firm glutes. Get ready to feel the burn in all the right places as you embark on this journey to strengthen and tone your lower body.

Building Powerful Legs

Quadriceps Dominance:

Let's kick things off by highlighting the mighty quadriceps, the muscles on the front of your thighs. Isometric exercises can effectively target these muscles, promoting strength and definition. The isometric wall sit is a classic example that requires no equipment.

Find a sturdy wall and lower yourself into a seated position, with your knees forming a 90-degree angle. Hold this position for as long as you can, feeling the burn in your quadriceps. This exercise not only strengthens your quads but also engages your core and glutes.

Hamstring Engagement:

For a well-rounded lower body workout, it's crucial to engage your hamstrings. Isometric hamstring curls can be performed using a stability ball. Lie on your back with your heels on the ball, lift your hips, and roll the ball towards you using your feet. Hold the fully contracted position, engaging your hamstrings, and then roll the ball back out. This exercise targets your hamstrings and glutes, fostering balance in your lower body muscle development.

Calf Definition:

Completing the trio of leg muscles, the calves deserve attention too. Isometric calf raises are an effective way to build definition in your calf muscles. Stand on the edge of a step, lift your heels, and hold the position for 10-15 seconds. This exercise not only targets your calf muscles but also enhances ankle stability.

Sculpting Firm Glutes

Glute Activation:

Now, let's shift our focus to sculpting those firm glutes that enhance your overall silhouette. Isometric glute bridges are a fantastic way to activate and strengthen your glute muscles. Lie on your back with your knees bent, lift your hips towards the ceiling, and hold the position. Squeeze your glutes at the top and feel the burn in your posterior chain. This exercise not only tones your glutes but also improves hip stability.

Lunges with a Twist:

Isometric lunges take the traditional lunge up a notch. Step forward into a lunge position, but instead of moving up and down, hold the lunge position for an extended period. This engages your glutes and quadriceps, providing a challenging yet effective workout for your lower body.

Inner and Outer Thighs:

To complete your lower body sculpting, consider isometric adductor and abductor exercises. Using a resistance band, perform side leg raises while standing to target your abductors. For adductors, sit on the floor with your legs extended and place the band around your ankles, then push your legs outward against the resistance. These exercises contribute to the sculpting of your inner and outer thighs, promoting a balanced lower body appearance.

Incorporating these lower body isometric exercises into your routine will not only build strength and definition in your legs and glutes but also improve overall lower body stability. Remember to listen to your body, start at a comfortable level, and gradually increase intensity as you progress on your fitness journey.

The power of isometric exercises extends beyond the perceived need for constant movement. By incorporating these upper and lower body isometric exercises into your routine, you are not only fostering strength and definition but also embracing a balanced and holistic approach to fitness. Consistency and dedication are the keys to unlocking the transformative changes that isometrics can bring to your body. So, take the plunge and embark on this journey to a stronger, more toned you!

Chapter 5: Personalizing Your Isometric Workout

Did you know that isometric exercises could be the key to reaching your fitness goals? In this chapter, we'll explore the power of customization and smooth integration. Whether you're aiming for strength, flexibility, or just want to add some spice to your routine, isometrics provide a flexible solution. Customize your workout to match your goals by blending static holds into your existing fitness routine. Get ready to see how this simple yet effective approach can enhance your fitness experience. Are you ready to unleash the potential of isometric exercises and reshape your workout plan?

Tailoring Workouts to Meet Your Goals

Isometric exercises, with their still contractions and gentle impact, are an excellent choice for women looking to adapt their fitness routines to specific goals. In this section, we'll explore the versatility of isometric exercises and how adjusting them to individual goals can improve your overall fitness journey.

Understanding Your Goals:

Before starting your isometric routine, it's vital to identify your fitness goals, whether it's building strength, improving posture, or managing stress. Isometric exercises cater to various goals, and by defining yours, you set the stage for a personalized and effective workout plan.

Building Strength and Tone:

If your main goal is to build strength and tone your muscles, isometric exercises provide a unique method. These exercises involve holding a static position, creating tension in specific muscle groups. For example, wall sits, planks, or static lunges can be included to engage major muscle groups, promoting strength development and definition.

When customizing your routine, consider the duration of each isometric hold. For those focusing on strength, shorter, more intense holds may be beneficial. It's about finding the right balance to challenge your muscles without compromising form.

Improving Endurance:

Isometric exercises can also be adapted to improve endurance. By extending the duration of each hold and incorporating a variety of positions, you can enhance your muscles' stamina. Gradually increasing hold times and including a mix of exercises like static squats, plank variations, and isometric push-ups will contribute to improved endurance over time.

Enhancing Flexibility:

Flexibility is another aspect that can be addressed through isometric exercises. While not as dynamic as some flexibility-focused routines, isometrics can help improve joint range of motion and overall flexibility. Incorporating positions that emphasize stretching and elongating muscles, such as isometric lunges or hamstring stretches, can contribute to increased flexibility over time.

Targeting Specific Areas:

One of the significant advantages of isometric exercises is their ability to target specific muscle groups. Tailor your routine to focus on areas that are particularly important to you. For example, if you want to strengthen your core, include isometric exercises like the plank or the boat pose. If you're looking to tone your arms, incorporate static holds like wall push-ups or bicep curls.

Customizing Intensity:

Another way to tailor isometric workouts is by adjusting the intensity. Beginners might start with shorter holds and fewer repetitions, gradually increasing as they become more comfortable. Advanced practitioners can challenge themselves with longer holds and more complex positions, ensuring continued progression aligned with their fitness goals.

Listen to Your Body:

While customization is crucial, it's equally important to listen to your body. If an exercise causes discomfort beyond the normal burn associated with isometrics, adjust accordingly or consult with a fitness professional. Every woman's body is unique, and the key to a successful isometric routine lies in finding the balance between challenge and comfort.

Tailoring isometric workouts to individual goals involves understanding what you want to achieve, selecting appropriate exercises, and customizing intensity and duration. By incorporating these personalized elements, you can make isometric exercises a powerful and enjoyable part of your fitness journey.

Now that we've explored tailoring isometric exercises to individual goals, let's look at seamlessly integrating these powerful static contractions into your current fitness routine. Whether you're a regular gym-goer, a yoga enthusiast, or someone with an established routine, adding isometrics can bring a new dimension to your fitness journey.

Isometrics as Additional Exercises:

Isometric exercises can serve as excellent additions to your current workout routine. For cardio enthusiasts, incorporating isometrics can strengthen muscles without excessive impact on joints, which is particularly helpful for high-impact activities like running or aerobics.

For those already engaged in strength training, isometrics provide a unique form of muscle engagement. By introducing static holds or isometric variations of traditional exercises, such as static lunges or isometric squats, you can target muscles differently, promoting overall strength and stability.

Integrating Isometrics into Yoga Practices:

Yoga practitioners can also benefit from including isometric exercises. While yoga naturally involves various static poses, adding specific isometric holds can intensify the practice. Including isometric variations of classic poses, like a static warrior pose or plank variations, can enhance the strength and stability aspects of your yoga routine.

Moreover, isometrics can enhance the mind-body connection that yoga emphasizes. Focusing on muscle engagement and breath control during isometric holds aligns well with the principles of mindfulness and concentration in yoga.

Blending Isometrics with Pilates:

For dedicated Pilates enthusiasts, integrating isometric exercises seamlessly complements the core-strengthening focus of this discipline. Adding static holds, such as an isometric bridge or plank, enhances core engagement, contributing to improved stability and balance. The controlled and precise movements inherent in Pilates align well with the deliberate nature of isometric exercises.

Creating Isometric Circuits:

Another effective way to incorporate isometrics into your existing routine is by creating dedicated isometric circuits. Designing a circuit that combines traditional exercises with isometric holds can provide a comprehensive workout. For example, pair dynamic movements like squats or lunges with static holds like wall sits or plank variations.

This approach not only keeps your routine dynamic and engaging but also ensures a well-rounded workout that addresses both dynamic and static muscle engagement.

Balancing Isometric and Dynamic Exercises:

Balance is key when incorporating isometrics into your current fitness routine. While isometrics offer unique benefits, they shouldn't replace dynamic movements entirely. Striking a balance between dynamic exercises and isometric holds ensures that you target muscles in various ways, promoting overall strength, flexibility, and endurance.

Progressive Integration:

If you're new to isometric exercises, consider progressively integrating them into your routine. Start with a few isometric holds per session and gradually increase the duration and intensity as your body adapts. This gradual incorporation allows your muscles and joints to acclimate to the static contractions, reducing the risk of overexertion.

Incorporating isometrics into your existing fitness routine offers a myriad of benefits, from enhanced muscle engagement to diversified workout routines. Whether you're a seasoned fitness enthusiast or just beginning your journey, isometric exercises can seamlessly become a valuable component of your overall wellness routine.

RECORD OBSERVATIONS/LESSONS HERE

____

____

____

____

____

____

____

____

Chapter 6: The Strength of Still Yoga

Did you know that combining simple yet powerful isometric exercises with yoga can change your fitness experience? Get ready for a big revelation in our next chapter - a smooth mix we call Still Yoga. Step into a place where muscles work with precision, traditional yoga poses get stronger, and quick workouts leave a lasting impression. Imagine gaining strength, flexibility, and mindfulness all at once. The secret is in the interesting blend waiting for you in the next pages. Brace yourself to uncover The Strength of Still Yoga and see your fitness routine change.

Blending Isometrics with Yoga Poses

Still Yoga is a strong mix of traditional isometric exercises and ancient yoga, creating a complete way to stay physically well. In this section, we'll explore the benefits that happen when isometrics combine with yoga poses, giving birth to what we lovingly call "The Strength of Still Yoga."

Isometric exercises mean squeezing specific muscles without changing their length or joint angle, providing a unique kind of resistance. This idea smoothly fits with the idea of yoga, which is about balance, flexibility, and mindfulness. Combining these two practices results in a workout that involves both the body and mind.

As you start your Still Yoga journey, you'll find that traditional yoga poses can be improved by adding isometric squeezes. For instance, during a classic yoga pose like Warrior II, squeezing your muscles while holding the pose can make it more intense, activating muscles more effectively.

The Strength of Still Yoga comes from its ability to target specific muscles with precision. By adding isometric squeezes to yoga poses, you not only make the workout more intense but also work your muscles in a way that traditional yoga alone might not. This focused effort can lead to better muscle tone and strength, helping you shape your body.

Moreover, blending isometrics with yoga improves stability and balance. Isometric squeezes make you activate and strengthen stabilizing muscles, fitting well with yoga's focus on balance. This combined approach helps you understand and control your body better.

One of the advantages of The Strength of Still Yoga is how efficient it is with time. Busy schedules often make it hard to exercise regularly, but Still Yoga offers a solution. The intensity of isometric squeezes allows for shorter but effective workouts. This means you can get the benefits of isometrics and yoga in a short time, making it easy to fit into your daily routine.

As you explore the world of Still Yoga, you'll notice a stronger connection between your mind and body. The mindfulness from traditional yoga is boosted by the focus needed during isometric squeezes. This syncing of breath, movement, and muscle engagement not only increases physical benefits but also reduces stress and promotes mental clarity.

The Strength of Still Yoga goes beyond regular exercise routines. It introduces a dynamic mix of isometric squeezes into the calm flow of yoga, resulting in a workout that not only improves strength and flexibility but also nurtures mindfulness and balance. As you embrace this mix, you'll find yourself on a journey to a healthier, more balanced you.

Boosting Flexibility and Strength Together

Welcome to Still Yoga, where the fusion of strength and flexibility takes the spotlight. In this section, we explore the amazing teamwork that happens when you improve both elements at the same time, offering a complete approach to staying physically well.

Flexibility and strength are often seen as opposites, but Still Yoga breaks down these barriers, showing they can work together. Traditional yoga is known for boosting flexibility with dynamic stretches and poses. On the other hand, isometric exercises focus on building strength by engaging muscles without movement. The magic occurs when these two practices come together.

Isometric squeezes in yoga poses create a unique challenge for your muscles. Take the Forward Fold, for example. By adding isometric squeezes, like pressing your palms together or engaging your core while holding the pose, you not only stretch more but also activate and strengthen the muscles. This dual action boosts both flexibility and strength, creating a more balanced and strong body.

The key to this double improvement is in proprioceptive neuromuscular facilitation (PNF). Still Yoga uses PNF principles by engaging a muscle group and then stretching it more during the relaxation phase. This communication improves flexibility and strengthens the muscles in their newly stretched state. The result is a dynamic interaction that benefits your body as a whole.

As you add isometrics to your yoga routine, you'll notice a big impact on joint stability. Isometric squeezes make you activate stabilizing muscles around joints, improving joint stability. This stability not only increases your overall range of motion but also lowers the risk of injuries, making your fitness experience safer and more effective.

Still Yoga's approach to boosting flexibility and strength goes beyond physical benefits. The focused engagement needed during isometric squeezes creates a deeper connection between your mind and body. As you move through poses with intentional muscle engagement, your awareness of your body's abilities and limits grows, leading to better body control.

Another great aspect of improving flexibility and strength together is the efficiency it brings to your workouts. Regular routines often separate flexibility and strength training sessions, demanding more time. Still Yoga simplifies this, offering a complete workout in a shorter time. This efficient approach makes it easier to fit into busy schedules while getting maximum results.

The fusion of flexibility and strength in Still Yoga offers a complete approach to fitness. By combining the dynamic stretches of yoga with the static intensity of isometric squeezes, you not only enhance your physical abilities but also nurture a deeper mind-body connection. Step into the world where flexibility and strength come together, and see the transformative power of Still Yoga in every stretch and squeeze.

"Transform your busy moments into powerful strides. Chapter 7 is your gateway to strength in simplicity – where quick isometric workouts become the catalyst for a robust, energized life. Busy women, seize the strength within the hustle!"

Chapter 7: 10-Minute Quick Workouts for Busy Women

Did you know that adding short bursts of still exercises to your busy day can bring excellent health benefits? In this chapter, we uncover the power of fast, focused still workouts for women on the move. Fact: Still exercises work many muscle groups without needing long sessions. Can just 10 minutes change your fitness routine? Get ready to find easy routines made for your life, offering a practical way to build strength, tone up, and boost energy. What if unlocking your body's abilities was easier than you thought? Let's explore the transformative impact of time-saving still exercises.

10-Minute Quick Workouts

Life can be busy, and finding time for a long exercise routine can be hard. However, with these quick still workouts, you can make big progress toward your fitness goals in just a bit of your day.

Still exercises mean contracting muscles without moving the joints, perfect for fast and effective workouts. The 10-minute length of these routines fits easily into your busy schedule, so you can focus on your health without losing valuable time.

Understanding Still Exercises

Before getting into the specific routines, let's quickly understand still exercises. Unlike regular exercises with repeated movements, still exercises focus on holding a position, promoting strength and endurance.

The good thing about still exercises is their flexibility. Whether you're at home, at work, or traveling, you can do these exercises without special equipment. This makes them an excellent choice for busy women without access to a gym or extended time for a workout.

The 10-Minute Still Routine

1. Warm-up (1 minute): Start with light cardio, like marching in place or gentle jumping jacks, to increase blood flow and prepare your muscles for the upcoming still exercises.

2. Wall Sit (2 minutes): Find a strong wall and slide down until your knees are bent at a 90-degree angle. Hold this position, working your quadriceps and glutes. This exercise is great for toning your lower body and building endurance.

3. Plank (2 minutes): Move to a plank position, supporting your body on your toes and forearms. Engage your core muscles, keeping your body in a straight line. Planks are excellent for strengthening your core and improving overall stability.

4. Chair Squats (2 minutes): Use a sturdy chair for controlled squats, lowering your body as if sitting down. Focus on working your leg muscles throughout the movement. Chair squats target your quads, hamstrings, and glutes.

5. Still Bicep Curl (2 minutes): Grab a pair of light dumbbells or household items. Hold them at shoulder height, elbows bent at a 90-degree angle. Keep this position, engaging your biceps. This exercise targets your arm muscles without complex movements.

Cool Down (1 minute): Finish the routine with gentle stretching to improve flexibility and help muscle recovery.

These 10-minute still workouts offer a quick yet effective solution for busy women wanting to add fitness to their daily lives. Focus on good form and controlled movements for the best results. Stay consistent, and you'll soon see the positive impact of these short but powerful sessions on your overall well-being.

Now, let's explore still exercises designed for quick office breaks. It's time to turn those sitting moments into chances to refresh your body and mind.

The Sitting Challenge

In today's fast work environment, it's common to find yourself sitting for a long time. Office jobs that involve sitting a lot can affect your health, causing issues like bad posture and muscle stiffness. However, with a few strategic still exercises, you can counteract the negative effects of sitting too long and add bursts of energy to your workday.

Benefits of Still Exercises during Office Breaks

Before we get into specific exercises, let's see why still exercises are perfect for your office routine. Isometrics let you work many muscle groups without needing much space or special equipment. You can discreetly add these exercises to your breaks, promoting circulation, reducing muscle tension, and boosting overall energy levels.

Office Break Still Routine

1. Desk Push-ups (2 minutes): Stand a few steps away from your desk, place your hands shoulder-width apart on the edge, and lean in. Lower your chest towards the desk and push back up. This push-up variation targets your chest, shoulders, and triceps.

2. Seated Leg Raise (2 minutes): While sitting at your desk, straighten one or both legs and hold in place for a few seconds. Lower the leg(s) back down without letting them touch the ground. This exercise engages your core and works your lower abdominal muscles.

3. Cubicle Wall Sit (2 minutes): Find an empty space against a cubicle wall and slide down into a sitting position with your knees at a 90-degree angle. This still squat engages your quadriceps and glutes, countering the effects of sitting too long.

4. Chair Dips (2 minutes): Using the edge of your office chair, position your hands on either side of your hips. Slide your bottom off the chair and lower your body, then push back up. Chair dips target your triceps and are excellent for toning your arms.

5. Still Neck Stretch (2 minutes): Gently tilt your head to one side, bringing your ear towards your shoulder, and hold the stretch for 30 seconds. Repeat on the other side. This exercise helps relieve tension in the neck and shoulders.

Adding Still Exercises to Your Workday

Consistency is vital to get the benefits of these office break still exercises. Try to add them to your daily routine, maybe during short breaks or even during virtual meetings where you can quietly do these movements. By doing this, you'll not only boost your physical well-being but also enhance mental clarity and productivity throughout your workday.

"Fuel your isometric fire with the right nutrition; a symphony of strength is composed not just in the gym but also in the choices you make at the table. Feed your body the building blocks of power, and watch as each isometric hold becomes a masterpiece of vitality."

Chapter 8: Eating Right and Isometric Exercise

Did you know that to get the most out of your isometric workouts, it's not just about how you move but also about what you eat and how you take care of your body? In this chapter, we'll explore the science behind how nutrition, staying hydrated, and recovery techniques can boost the effectiveness of isometric training, especially for women. From the importance of having a good mix of proteins, carbs, and fats to keeping your muscles hydrated, we'll share practical tips to make your isometric exercises even better. Get ready to learn the essential basics that will help you fuel your body efficiently and improve your outcomes in isometric exercises.

Success in isometric exercises isn't just about the physical effort; it's also about giving your body the proper fuel for better performance and results. In this part, we'll discuss the vital link between what you eat and isometric training, guiding you on how to fuel your body for success in your isometric activities.

Understanding the Connection between Nutrition and Isometric Training

Isometric exercises need a special mix of muscle strength and endurance. While doing these static contractions, your muscles need a continuous energy source to perform well. Good nutrition is essential to provide this energy and support your muscles during isometric exercises.

Balanced Nutrients

Make sure your diet includes a mix of proteins, carbs, and fats. Proteins help in muscle repair and growth, carbs give the energy needed for isometric contractions, and healthy fats contribute to overall body functions.

Protein for Muscle Health

Proteins are crucial for anyone doing isometric exercises because they build and repair muscles. Include lean protein sources like poultry, fish, tofu, and legumes in your diet. These foods help your muscles recover after challenging isometric sessions.

Using Carbs as Energy

Carbs are the main energy source for your body, especially during intense activities like isometric exercises. Choose complex carbs like whole grains, fruits, and vegetables for a steady release of energy, helping you sustain your workout. This sustained energy is crucial for holding isometric contractions over a long period.

Staying Hydrated and Electrolytes

Keeping hydrated is vital for optimal performance in isometric exercises. Water is essential for overall health and helps maintain muscle function and joint flexibility. Also, consider replenishing lost electrolytes, especially during intense isometric routines. Drinks with electrolytes or natural sources like coconut water can help restore the balance.

Meal Timing and Isometric Workouts

When you eat can significantly impact your isometric training. Having a balanced meal a few hours before your session ensures your body has the nutrients it needs. Also, a post-workout meal with protein and carbs helps with muscle recovery and restores energy.

Pre-Workout Eating

Eat a light meal with both carbs and proteins about 2-3 hours before your isometric workout. This provides a steady release of energy during your session, preventing fatigue.

Post-Workout Eating

After your isometric routine, aim for a post-workout meal or snack within the first hour. This should include both proteins and carbs to kickstart muscle recovery and replenish glycogen stores.

To sum up, the connection between nutrition and isometric training is crucial. Choosing the right nutrients at the right time not only boosts your performance during isometric exercises but also supports muscle recovery and overall well-being. Make thoughtful choices in your diet, stay hydrated, and witness your isometric success as your body gets the optimal fuel it needs.

Hydration and recovery play vital roles in a successful isometric training plan. Ensuring your body gets enough fluids and using effective recovery strategies can make a big difference in your overall performance and well-being. Let's explore why hydration and recovery matter in the context of isometric exercises.

Hydration Essentials for Isometric Success

Understanding Fluid Balance

Hydration isn't just about quenching your thirst; it's about maintaining the right balance of fluids in your body. This balance is critical for isometric exercises. When you do static contractions, your muscles generate heat, and proper hydration helps dissipate this heat, preventing overheating and promoting optimal muscle function.

Water as the Foundation

Water is the main element for hydration, and its importance can't be overstated. It lubricates joints, transports nutrients to cells, and helps regulate body temperature – all crucial for successful isometric training. Aim to drink water consistently throughout the day, not just during your workout.

Individual Hydration Needs

The amount of water you need can vary based on factors like body weight, climate, and the intensity of your isometric routine. A general guideline is to consume at least eight 8-ounce glasses of water a day, but individual needs may differ. Listen to your body – if you feel thirsty, drink, and pay attention to your urine color, aiming for a pale yellow shade.

Effective Hydration Strategies during Isometric Workouts

Sip, Don't Guzzle

Rather than drinking a lot of water at once, sip it throughout your isometric workout. This prevents overloading your stomach and minimizes the risk of discomfort. Small, regular sips ensure a steady intake, keeping you adequately hydrated without causing digestive issues during your exercises.

Balancing Electrolytes

In addition to water, pay attention to your electrolyte balance, especially if you sweat a lot during isometric exercises. Electrolytes like sodium, potassium, and magnesium are crucial for muscle contraction and fluid balance. Consider including electrolyte-rich beverages or snacks, especially if your workouts are long or intense.

Post-Workout Hydration

Rehydrating after your isometric session is equally important. Your body loses fluids through sweat during exercise, and replenishing these lost fluids is essential for recovery. Aim to consume water or a hydrating beverage within the first hour after your workout to support the recovery process.

Prioritizing Recovery for Optimal Isometric Results

Understanding the Importance of Recovery

Isometric exercises put a lot of stress on your muscles, and prioritizing recovery is key to preventing fatigue, minimizing soreness, and getting the most out of your workouts. Incorporate effective recovery strategies into your routine to ensure your muscles are ready for the next isometric challenge.

Quality Sleep for Muscle Repair

One of the most important aspects of recovery is getting good sleep. During sleep, your body releases growth hormone, which is crucial for muscle repair and growth. Aim for 7-9 hours of uninterrupted sleep each night to optimize your body's recovery processes.

Active Recovery Techniques

Engage in light, low-impact activities on your rest days to enhance blood flow and promote muscle recovery. Activities like walking, swimming, or gentle stretching can help reduce muscle stiffness and improve overall flexibility.

Nutrient-Rich Post-Workout Snacks

Support your muscles by eating nutrient-rich snacks after your workout. A mix of protein and carbs helps replenish glycogen stores and kickstarts the muscle repair process. Greek yogurt with fruits, a protein smoothie, or a handful of nuts and dried fruits are excellent choices.

Include Stretching and Foam Rolling

Add dynamic stretches and foam rolling to your post-workout routine to enhance flexibility and ease muscle tightness. These practices contribute to improved range of motion and reduce the risk of injury during your isometric exercises.

To conclude, hydration and recovery are crucial elements of a successful isometric training journey. Prioritize proper hydration, adopt effective recovery strategies, and see how your body responds positively to these supportive measures. By making these practices a part of your routine, you set the stage for improved performance, reduced muscle soreness, and overall success in your isometric pursuits.

Chapter 9: Unveiling the Relationship between Mind and Body through Isometric Exercises

Did you ever consider that the key to cultivating a healthier mind might lie in the intensity of your muscle contractions? In this ninth installment of our exploration into Isometric Exercises for Women, we will unravel the intricate connection between the mind and body. Brace yourself for a profound revelation: the subtle art of isometrics, when combined with mindful practices such as meditation, has the potential not only to alleviate stress but also to elevate focus and mental well-being. Can the power to reduce stress and enhance concentration truly be found within the world of isometric exercises? Let's delve into the intricacies of this fascinating connection and uncover the transformative impact it can have on your overall well-being.

Within the scope of isometric exercises for women, the symbiotic relationship between the mind and body plays a pivotal role in achieving holistic well-being. In this section, we will delve into the profound impact of incorporating meditation into isometric exercises.

Understanding the Harmony between Mind and Body

The fusion of meditation and isometric exercises creates a powerful synergy that transcends the physical realm. Isometric exercises involve contracting muscles without changing their length, promoting both strength and endurance. Simultaneously, meditation cultivates a serene mental state, fostering emotional balance and mindfulness.

Unveiling the Mental Benefits

1. Stress Reduction: Isometric exercises, when accompanied by meditation, act as a formidable stress-relief duo. Stress often manifests physically, causing muscle tension and discomfort. Engaging in isometrics while maintaining a meditative mindset alleviates stress by promoting muscle relaxation and mental tranquility.

2. Enhanced Focus: Meditation enhances concentration, a skill directly applicable to isometric exercises. The mindful approach during isometrics helps you focus on the specific muscle groups being engaged, refining your mind-muscle connection. This heightened awareness contributes to better form, increased efficiency, and improved results.

The How-To of Meditative Isometrics

1. Setting the Scene: Find a quiet space where you can perform your isometric exercises without distractions. Begin with a few deep breaths to center yourself and transition into a meditative state.

2. Mindful Muscle Engagement: As you proceed with isometric exercises, concentrate on the targeted muscle group. Picture the muscle working, contracting, and releasing. This mental imagery not only deepens your connection with your body but also intensifies the effectiveness of the exercises.

3. Breath Awareness: Sync your breath with your isometric movements. Inhale during the muscle contraction phase and exhale during the relaxation phase. This rhythmic breathing not only enhances oxygen flow to the muscles but also promotes a calming effect on your nervous system.

The Scientific Backing

Research has shown that combining isometric exercises with meditation induces positive changes in the brain. The dual impact on the mind and body helps reduce cortisol levels, the hormone associated with stress. Additionally, the release of endorphins, triggered by both activities, contributes to an overall sense of well-being.

Incorporating Meditation into Your Routine

To embrace the fusion of meditation and isometric exercises, consider dedicating a few minutes to mindfulness before or after your workout sessions. Experiment with different meditation techniques, such as guided imagery or mindfulness meditation, to discover what resonates best with you.

By intertwining these practices, you not only sculpt a stronger physique but also nurture a resilient and serene mind. As you embark on this transformative journey, remember that the path to wellness involves the harmonious balance of both body and mind.

Unraveling the Benefits: Stress Reduction and Improved Focus

In the pursuit of overall well-being through isometric exercises for women, Chapter 9.2 delves deeper into the profound impact these exercises have on stress reduction and focus improvement. The interconnectedness between physical activity and mental clarity forms a cornerstone for achieving a balanced and fulfilling lifestyle.

The Stress-Reduction Power of Isometric Exercises

1. Muscle Relaxation: Isometric exercises inherently involve contracting muscles without joint movement, leading to muscle relaxation. This physical release of tension extends beyond the muscles, influencing the nervous system to unwind. As a result, the practice of isometrics becomes a therapeutic remedy for the accumulated stress of daily life.

2. Cortisol Regulation: Isometric exercises play a crucial role in regulating cortisol, the body's primary stress hormone. Engaging in these exercises prompts the release of endorphins, which counteract the effects of cortisol. This hormonal equilibrium contributes to a more serene mental state, fostering resilience against stressors.

Improved Focus through Isometric Exercises

1. Mind-Muscle Connection: Isometric exercises demand a heightened awareness of the muscles being engaged. This intentional focus on specific muscle groups enhances the mind-muscle connection, sharpening your concentration during workouts. The deliberate mental engagement in each exercise cultivates a sense of mindfulness, redirecting your attention away from external stressors.

2. Neuroplasticity Enhancement: Regular isometric exercises stimulate neuroplasticity – the brain's ability to adapt and reorganize. This adaptability extends to cognitive functions, including attention and focus. As you consistently engage in isometrics, your brain forms new neural connections that contribute to improved concentration and cognitive flexibility.

Implementing Stress Reduction and Improved Focus in Your Routine

1. Structured Workouts: Incorporate isometric exercises strategically within your workout routine. Begin with a warm-up to prepare your muscles, then seamlessly transition into isometrics. As you progress, pay mindful attention to the sensation in each muscle group, allowing the exercises to become a mindful practice.

2. Progressive Relaxation: Integrate progressive muscle relaxation techniques into your post-workout routine. After completing isometric exercises, consciously release any lingering tension in each muscle group. This intentional relaxation aids in the physical recovery process and contributes to an overall sense of calm.

Scientific Validation of Stress Reduction and Focus Improvement

Numerous studies substantiate the stress-reducing and focus-improving benefits of isometric exercises. The physiological responses, including lowered cortisol levels and increased endorphin release, align with a reduction in perceived stress. Moreover, brain imaging studies showcase the positive impact of isometrics on neural pathways associated with attention and concentration.

In the grand tapestry of achieving optimal well-being, isometric exercises, when harmoniously combined with meditation, emerge as a potent elixir for both body and mind. As we navigate through the multifaceted landscape of mind-body connections, it becomes evident that the realm of isometric exercises holds untold potential for transformative change. This journey towards holistic wellness invites you to embrace the unity of physical and mental practices, unlocking a path to a resilient, focused, and serene existence. So, as you embark on this exploration, remember that every contraction and every moment of mindful awareness contributes to the masterpiece of your overall well-being.

Chapter 10: Progress Tracking and Adjusting Goals

In this chapter, we will delve into the multifaceted aspects of tracking your fitness progress and making necessary adjustments to your isometric exercise routine for optimal results. The journey to a healthier you involves more than just the physical exertion of sweating it out; it's about understanding the importance of the process within each pose. Join us in unlocking the secrets of sustainable progress and continuous improvement in your fitness endeavors.

Importance of Tracking Fitness Progress

Commencing a fitness journey is a commendable decision, especially for women engaged in isometric exercises. Understanding the significance of tracking progress becomes a pivotal aspect of achieving health and fitness goals. Monitoring your journey not only serves as a motivational factor but also provides valuable insights into your body's response to isometric exercises.

Why is tracking progress essential?

1. Motivation Boost:

The act of tracking your fitness progress acts as a constant motivator. Witnessing tangible improvements, such as an increase in the duration of holding isometric poses or enhanced muscle tone, reinforces your commitment and fuels the desire to push further.

2. Goal Assessment:

 It serves as a compass for assessing your initial goals. By regularly evaluating your progress, you can determine if your isometric exercise routine aligns with your objectives. This allows for necessary adjustments, ensuring that your efforts are directed towards realistic and achievable milestones.

3. Identification of Plateaus:

Even the most effective fitness programs can reach plateaus. Tracking progress helps identify these plateaus, enabling you to tweak your isometric exercises or introduce variations to overcome stagnation. Plateau awareness is crucial for maintaining a consistent trajectory towards your fitness aspirations.

4. Prevention of Overtraining:

Isometric exercises, while highly beneficial, can lead to overtraining if not managed properly. Monitoring your progress allows you to recognize signs of overtraining, such as persistent fatigue or decreased performance. Adjusting your routine in response to these indicators ensures a healthier and sustainable fitness journey.

5. Health Metrics Monitoring:

Beyond the aesthetic aspects, tracking progress allows you to monitor essential health metrics. This includes improvements in cardiovascular health, increased flexibility, and enhanced overall well-being. These holistic benefits are equally important in gauging the success of your isometric exercise routine.

How to track progress effectively:

1. Keep a Workout Journal:

Maintaining a workout journal serves as a comprehensive record of your isometric exercises. Note down details such as the duration of each pose, any modifications made, and how your body feels post-workout. This provides a tangible reference for evaluating your progress over time.

2. Use Technology:

Leverage fitness apps and wearable devices to track key metrics. Many apps allow you to log your isometric workouts, monitor heart rate, and track changes in body composition. These tools provide a visual representation of your journey and make it easier to identify patterns and trends.

3. Regular Assessments:

Incorporate regular assessments into your routine. Periodically evaluate your strength, flexibility, and endurance. These assessments act as checkpoints, allowing you to celebrate achievements and make informed decisions about adjusting your isometric exercise program.

The importance of tracking fitness progress in your isometric exercise journey cannot be overstated. It not only keeps you motivated but also serves as a dynamic tool for optimizing your routine, preventing setbacks, and ensuring a fulfilling and sustainable path to improved health and wellness.

Modifying Isometric Programs for Continuous Improvement

As you progress on this empowering journey, the ability to modify your isometric programs becomes an invaluable tool for ensuring continuous improvement and addressing your evolving fitness needs. This section will delve into why and how you can tailor your isometric exercises for optimal results.

Why modify isometric programs?

1. Adaptation to Strength Gains:

As you consistently engage in isometric exercises, your muscles adapt and become stronger. Modifying your program allows you to progressively challenge your muscles, preventing them from plateauing. Gradually increasing the intensity or duration of your poses ensures continued strength gains.

2. Addressing Weaknesses:

Isometric exercises target specific muscle groups. Modifying your program enables you to identify and address any muscle imbalances or weaknesses. By incorporating variations that target underdeveloped areas, you create a more well-rounded and effective fitness routine.

3. Preventing Boredom:

Exercise adherence is more likely when routines remain engaging and enjoyable. Introducing variations in your isometric exercises not only prevents boredom but also keeps your mind actively engaged during workouts. This psychological aspect is crucial for maintaining long-term commitment to your fitness journey.

4. Injury Prevention:

Modifying your program helps in avoiding overuse injuries. If certain muscles or joints are consistently strained, adjusting your routine to provide those areas with adequate rest or incorporating alternative exercises can prevent overuse injuries and promote overall joint health.

How to modify isometric programs effectively:

1. Progressive Overload:

Adopt a principle of progressive overload by gradually increasing the intensity of your isometric exercises. This could involve holding poses for a longer duration, increasing the number of repetitions, or incorporating advanced variations. This method challenges your muscles, promoting continuous improvement.

2. Incorporate Dynamic Movements:

While isometric exercises focus on static muscle contractions, incorporating dynamic movements adds variety to your routine. For example, combining isometric holds with dynamic movements like leg lifts or arm reaches enhances muscle engagement and overall effectiveness.

3. Explore Different Angles:

Modify your isometric exercises by experimenting with different angles and positions. Changing the angle of a pose alters the emphasis on specific muscles, providing a more comprehensive workout and addressing any muscle imbalances.

4. Vary Duration and Frequency:

Adjust the duration and frequency of your isometric exercises based on your fitness goals. Shorter, more intense sessions may target muscle endurance, while longer holds can focus on strength development. Periodically changing the frequency adds a layer of variability to your routine.

5. Listen to Your Body:

Pay close attention to how your body responds to different modifications. If you experience discomfort or strain, it's essential to listen to your body and make adjustments accordingly. Gradual progression is key to avoiding injuries and ensuring a sustainable fitness journey.

By adapting to strength gains, addressing weaknesses, preventing boredom, and incorporating varied approaches, you'll maximize the effectiveness of your isometric exercises and experience a more fulfilling and evolving fitness journey. Keep challenging yourself, stay attuned to your body, and celebrate the continuous progress you make along the way!

Conclusion

As we conclude this exercise adventure, I want to thank you sincerely for joining me on this path to a stronger and healthier you. Your dedication has not gone unnoticed. Every isometric hold, every adjustment, and every achievement reflects your strength and determination.

You've put time and effort into shaping a version of yourself that exudes strength and vitality. Your journey is ongoing; it's a continuous exploration of your potential. Whether you're a beginner or a dedicated enthusiast, your commitment to well-being is motivating.

I encourage you to explore more in our shared health and fitness world. Check out other books by this author to learn about various aspects of a healthy lifestyle. Your feedback is important; leave reviews, share your experiences, and inspire others on their transformative paths.

As you close this chapter, carry the strength you've built, the knowledge you've gained, and the resilience you've shown. Your body shows what consistent effort and a positive mindset can achieve. Until we meet again, stay active, stay healthy, and continue embracing the amazing journey of self-improvement. Thank you, and may your future chapters bring even greater achievements and well-being.

BONUS

Isometric Exercise Secrets for Women Workout Journal

Welcome to the EmpowerHER Workout Journal — your dedicated companion on the transformative journey to a stronger, healthier you. This bonus journal is designed to enhance your experience with "EmpowerHER: The Ultimate Guide to Isometric Mastery for Women." Utilize these practical tools to track your progress, set goals, and celebrate your victories along the way.

Date: ______________

EXER	SETS	REPS	DURATION	INTENSITY (1-10)	NOTES
UPPER BODY ISOMETRICS					
LOWER BODY ISOMETRICS					
YOGA FUSION					
QUICK WORKOUTS					

Goal Tracker

Short-Term Goals:

1. _______________________________________

2. _______________________________________

3. _______________________________________

Long-Term Goals:

1. _______________________________________

2. _______________________________________

3. _______________________________________

Today's Meals:

MEAL	FOOD ITEMS	WATER INTAKE (OZ)	NOTES
Breakfast			
Snack			
Lunch			
Snack			
Dinner			

Highlight of the Week:

____

____

____

____

Challenges Faced:

____

____

____

____

How I Overcame Challenges:

____

____

____

____

____

Self-Reflection and Gratitudes:

____

____

____

____

Conclusion:

This Workout Journal is your personal space for triumphs, challenges, and growth. Use it consistently, and watch your journey unfold. Celebrate your achievements, learn from setbacks, and embrace the strength within. Your transformation starts here.

NOTE: You can print out as many copies of this workout journal as you want for more daily inputs and records.